I Speak Life:(Seeking The Great Physician)

Kim Ruff-Moore

Published by Ruff Moore Media, 2024.

I SPEAK LIFE:(SEEKING THE GREAT PHYSICIAN)

First edition. February 22, 2024.

Copyright © 2024 Kim Ruff-Moore.

ISBN: 979-8224203888

Written by Kim Ruff-Moore.

Dedication

To the memory of my mother Sara Nell Lane, My Grandmother Carrie and my Aunt Thurlie Mae

Continue to Rest Well until Christ returns .

TABLE OF CONTENTS

Introduction

The story of my family's battle with cancer was at one time a heavy burden I carried. My mother, grandmother, and aunt all fell victim to this dreadful disease called cancer. Breast and ovarian cancer to be exact and they leave behind a legacy of uncertainty. According to science, I am at a higher risk of facing the same fate. The numbers don't lie, painting a grim picture of my future. Yet, I refuse to let statistics define my destiny. Instead, I cling to hope and faith, believing in something greater than the odds stacked against me. I find comfort in the words of Jeremiah 29:11, trusting in God's plan for my life and holding onto the promise of a brighter tomorrow.

I turn to God as my source of healing and strength. I know that true healing can only come from Him. With every prayer, I speak out against the disease that threatens to consume me, asking God to break the cycle of sickness that has plagued my family for generations. I do not have breast cancer and I ask God to remove the possibility from my path. I boldly come to God asking Him to not allow it to be my portion. I intervene on behalf of my beautiful sisters and ask God to shield them and protect them as well. I seek to break this generational curse. I know that God has already equipped me so I exercise my faith and boldly seek His face daily to cover us and protect us. To my friends who are battling this disease I ask God to heal them and bless them indeed.

Though the road ahead may be difficult, I walk with determination and resilience. I refuse to let fear dictate my life, choosing instead to place my trust in God's unfailing love and mercy. And as I continue on this journey, I am filled with hope, knowing that I am not alone in this fight against cancer.

BREAKING THE GENERATIONAL CURSE

I have had people say that losing my mom, grandma, and aunt to this awful disease casts a shadow over my own health. Science says I'm more likely to face the same fate. It's scary, no denying that. I am human, so I will be the first to admit that it takes faith and trusting God on a daily basis.

I'm not letting statistics dictate my future. I'm holding onto hope, trusting there's something bigger than these odds against me. Jeremiah 29:11 gives me peace, reminding me that God has plans for me, plans for good things, not for disaster. I believe that God has given us the ability to speak into our lives and our destiny.

When things feel uncertain, I turn to God for strength and mental as well as physical healing. I know He's the ultimate healer. Every prayer I say is a plea to break the cycle of sickness that's plagued my family.

Even though the road ahead is a faith and prayer walk , I'm not giving in to fear. I'm leaning on God's love and mercy to get me through. And I'm not alone in this fight. My loved ones and community are here for me, cheering me on and praying for me.

Taking care of my health is a priority too. Eating well, staying active, and keeping up with check-ups are all part of the plan. Prevention and early detection are key.

But beyond these practical steps, I cling to the belief that sickness isn't what God wants for us. He desires for us to be whole and healthy. In John 10:10, Jesus says He came to give us life in abundance. And in 3 John 1:2, it's written that God wishes above all things for us to prosper and be in good health. That's His promise, and I choose to believe it because God doesn't lie.

So, I'm asking God to cover me and bless me, to keep sickness and disease away from me and my family. I'm even taking it a step further by addressing what could be a generational curse in my family. The premature deaths from cancer seem like a pattern, a curse that tries to snatch away the women in my family before their time. But I denounce that curse. I refuse to accept it as my fate. Instead, I'm aligning my health with God's Word, believing for His divine protection and healing.

In breaking generational curses, I find strength in the scripture. In Exodus 34:7, it's written that God "visits the iniquity of the fathers on the children and the children's children, to the third and the fourth generation." But in Galatians 3:13, it says, "Christ redeemed us from the curse of the law by becoming a curse for us." This means that through Jesus Christ, we have the power to break free from generational curses. With His sacrifice, we can claim victory over every curse that seeks to bind us.

So, armed with faith and empowered by scripture, I march forward, breaking free from the chains of sickness and claiming the abundant life that God has promised me.

Breaking generational curses means speaking life and claiming victory over the sickness and death that have plagued my family. In this journey, I've learned the power of words. Proverbs 18:21 says, "The tongue has the power of life and death." So, I choose to speak life into my situation, rejecting fear and embracing God's promise of healing.

I won't accept the idea that sickness and early death are our family's destiny. Instead, I boldly declare Isaiah 53:5, believing that "by His wounds, we are healed." It's not just wishful thinking; it's trusting in God's truth.

I also know the importance of breaking ties with past patterns. In Jesus' name, I cut any links to sickness and suffering in my family history. I refuse to let the past define my future, trusting in God's freedom and victory.

Romans 8:37 reminds me that "in all these things, we are more than conquerors." I'm not a victim; I'm empowered by God's love.

With each step, I embrace my identity as God's child, meant for health and wholeness. Though it was scary initially, I trust in God's faithfulness.

So, breaking generational curses isn't just about actions; it's a spiritual battle fought with faith and prayer. As I speak life and claim victory, I believe in God's promise to lead me to a future filled with hope and restoration.

I wish I could say that I have all the answers and that speaking life into a breast cancer diagnosis guarantees healing. I wish I could offer a foolproof solution, a magic cure that erases all pain and suffering. But the truth is, life doesn't always unfold according to our desires, and healing is not always immediate or apparent.

What I do know, however, is the power of faith and the strength that comes from believing in something greater than ourselves. For me, that source of strength is my faith in God. I've seen firsthand the miracles that can happen when we surrender our fears and doubts and place our trust in Him.

God has promised us life and death are in the power of the tongue, and while that may not always translate into physical healing, it does offer us a sense of control over our circumstances. Through prayer and relationship with Him, we have the power to break generational curses and overcome the obstacles that stand in our way.

I believe in Jehovah Rapha, our healer, the Great Physician who can mend even the deepest wounds. I've witnessed the transformative power of His love and mercy, and I know that by the stripes of Jesus Christ, we are healed.

But healing isn't always about the physical body. Sometimes, it's about finding peace and acceptance in the midst of pain and suffering. It's about trusting in God's plan, even when it doesn't make sense to us.

I've learned that we have the authority to speak life into our situations, to declare victory over our struggles, and to claim the promises of God for our lives. The power of life and death is in the power of the tongue, and when we speak words of faith and hope, we invite miracles to unfold in our lives.

So, while I may not have all the answers, I take comfort in knowing that I serve a God who is bigger than any diagnosis, stronger than any illness, and more loving than I could ever imagine. And with Him by my side, I can face whatever challenges come my way, knowing that I am never alone.

It is not about the outcome but about the journey – the lessons we learn, the people we meet, and the faith that sustains us through it all. And for that, I am eternally grateful.

As I reflect on my mother's journey and my own faith, I'm reminded of the countless others who have faced similar battles. Breast cancer doesn't discriminate; it affects people of all ages, races, and backgrounds. And while the road to healing may be fraught with obstacles, I've seen the incredible resilience of the human spirit.

I've met warriors who have looked cancer in the face and refused to back down, who have found strength in the midst of their struggles and hope in the darkest of moments. Their stories inspire me to keep pushing forward, to never lose faith in the power of prayer and the promise of healing.

But I also recognize that not everyone receives the miracle they so desperately seek. Some are called home far too soon, their lives cut short by a disease that knows no mercy. And in those moments of heartbreak and loss, it can be difficult to reconcile our faith with the harsh realities of life.

Yet even in the midst of our pain, I believe there is beauty to be found. For it is in our brokenness that we find strength, in our vulnerability that we find connection, and in our grief that we find compassion. And though we may never fully understand why some are healed while others are not, we can take solace in the knowledge that we serve a God who is always present, always loving, and always faithful.

So, as I continue on my own journey of faith and mental healing, I hold onto the words of Scripture: "For I know the plans I have for you, declares the Lord, plans to prosper you and not to harm you, plans to give you hope and a future" (Jeremiah 29:11). And with each step I take, I trust that God is guiding me, protecting me, and leading me toward a future filled with hope and promise.

In the end, it's not about the number of days we have on this earth, but about the impact we make and the legacy we leave behind. My mother may have lost her battle with breast cancer, but her spirit lives on in the lives of those she touched, a testament to the power of love, faith, and resilience.

And so, I continue to speak life into my circumstances, knowing that God is with me every step of the way. For with Him, all things are possible, and even in the midst of life's greatest challenges, there is always hope.

LOSING MY MOTHER

Losing my mother to breast cancer is a wound that has never fully healed. Even after all these years, the memories are still vivid, etched into my mind like photographs in an album. She was a remarkable woman, one who faced her illness with courage and grace, despite the immense burden it placed upon her.

I remember the day she told me as if it were yesterday. She was only 35 at the time, too young to be confronted with such a devastating illness. But true to her nature, she remained stoic, shielding us from the full weight of her fears and worries.

My mother was always a private person, keeping her struggles close to her heart. Even as she battled the disease, she rarely spoke about it, preferring to bear the burden silently. It wasn't until I stumbled upon literature about breast cancer around the house that I began to piece together the gravity of her situation. The signs were there in her bedroom and bathroom – remnants of surgeries and treatments that she never openly discussed.

Her own mother's battle with ovarian cancer cast a long shadow over my mother's life. Losing her own mother at such a young age had left scars that never fully healed. I could sense the weight of that loss in her, the unspoken fear that she too would leave her children behind, just as her mother had done.

When she went into the hospital for what she called a lumpectomy, I knew deep down that it was more than just a routine procedure. The fear hung heavy in the air, suffocating us all with its presence. And when the cancer returned, more aggressive than ever, it felt like a cruel twist of fate.

I was living in Chattanooga, four hours away from her, when she received the devastating news. But by the grace of God , I was able to take time off from work and spend an entire week with her over Christmas. It was a bittersweet reunion, seeing her so thin and frail, yet still radiating with the same beauty and strength that had always defined her.

Those precious moments together are etched into my memory, a beacon of light in the darkness that followed. We laughed, we cried, and we shared memories that will stay with me forever. But even as we clung to each other, I could feel the inevitable looming on the horizon.

Less than a year after her diagnosis, my mother was gone. The cancer had spread with a merciless speed, attacking her body with a ferocity that left us all reeling. In the end, she was just 52 years old, taken from us far too soon.

Her passing left a void in our lives that can never be filled. But in the midst of the pain and sorrow, I find solace in the memories we shared and the lessons she taught us. She may be gone, but her spirit lives on in each of us, a guiding light in the darkness of our grief.

And so, I carry her with me always, a silent presence in my heart that gives me strength in the face of life's greatest challenges. She may have lost her battle with cancer, but her legacy lives on in the lives of her children and grandchildren. And for that, I am eternally grateful.

My mother's battle with breast cancer wasn't just a personal struggle; it was a testament to the resilience of the human spirit. Despite the pain and uncertainty, she never lost her sense of self or her unwavering love for her family.

As her illness progressed, I watched in awe as she faced each new challenge with unwavering courage. She refused to let cancer define her, clinging to the things that brought her joy – her family, her faith, and the simple pleasures of life.

But as much as she tried to shield us from the harsh realities of her illness, I could see the toll it took on her. The fear that lurked behind her eyes, the weariness that settled into her bones – it was a constant reminder of the fragility of life.

In those final days, I was unable to gather around her bedside. I was unaware of the reality that she would actually leave us and fall asleep in Jesus. Despite the pain and the uncertainty, she faced death with a quiet dignity that left us all in awe.

And when she finally slipped away, with my dad by her side, it felt like the end of an era. But even in death, her legacy lives on, a beacon of hope and inspiration for all who knew her.

In the years since her passing, I've often found myself turning to her memory for strength and guidance. In moments of doubt or despair, I can feel her presence beside me, urging me to keep moving forward, to never give up hope.

And so, I carry her with me always, especially when I look in the mirror. I look so much like her now. Though she may be gone, her spirit lives on in the hearts of those who loved her, a reminder that even in our darkest moments, there is always light to be found.

In the end, my mother's battle with breast cancer was not just a tragedy; it was a triumph of the human spirit. And though she may have lost her life to the disease, she will always be remembered for the strength, courage, and love that defined her.

THIS BATTLE IS PERSONAL

The battle against breast cancer, or cancer in general, is deeply personal for me. Despite the grim statistics and data that suggest I am predisposed to this disease due to my genes and the fate of my mother and grandmother, I refuse to accept it as my destiny. This fight is not just about me; it's about my four beloved biological sisters whom I cherish dearly and want to see live long, healthy lives. It's about my seven nieces, whom I want to experience life's joys without the shadow of this illness looming over them. At 52, the same age my mother lost her battle, I am reminded of the urgency to fight for my own life. I have a loving husband, a soulmate, with whom I've been blessed to share nearly two years of marriage. I have a 22-year-old son who still needs me, and I have so much more life to live. This is deeply personal; it's about speaking life into the face of statistical probability. I declare that I will live and not die, trusting in the healing touch of the Great Physician, Jehovah Rapha, to align my health with His word.

This battle against breast cancer, or any form of cancer, isn't just about defying statistics or relying solely on medical science. It's about embracing faith, hope, and the power of resilience. My journey is intertwined with the lives of those I love – my family, my husband, my son. Their love fuels my determination to fight, to cling onto every moment, and to envision a future where cancer isn't a looming threat. I refuse to let fear dictate my narrative. Instead, I choose to speak life into existence, to trust in the divine intervention of a higher power. I believe in the possibility of miracles, in the capacity of my body to heal, and in the unwavering support of my community. This is a battle that extends beyond the physical realm; it's a test of faith, perseverance, and unwavering resolve.

As I proceed on this journey, I draw strength from the stories of survivors, the comforting embrace of loved ones, and the steadfast hope that tomorrow holds. Every day is a testament to the resilience of the human spirit, a reminder that even in the darkest of times, there is light waiting to be found. So yes, this battle is personal – but it's also a testament to the power of love, faith, and the indomitable human spirit. The battle against breast cancer, or any form of cancer, isn't just about defying statistics or relying solely on medical science. It's about embracing faith, hope, and the power of resilience. My journey is intertwined with the lives of those I love – my family, my husband, our children. Their love fuels my determination to fight and speak life.

At the heart of this battle lies the intricate interplay between science and spirituality, between empirical data and the unseen forces that govern our existence. On one hand, there's the stark reality of genetic predisposition, of statistical probabilities that seem to foretell an inevitable fate. But on the other hand, there's the undeniable power of belief, of speaking life into existence, and of trusting in the healing touch of a higher power.

For me, this battle took on a deeply personal dimension at the age of 52, the same age my mother succumbed to her illness. It was a sobering reminder of mortality, of the fragility of life, and of the urgency to seize every moment with unwavering determination. But amidst the fear and uncertainty, there was also a profound sense of purpose – a resolve to defy the odds, to rewrite the narrative, and to emerge stronger and more resilient than ever before.

My family, comprising four biological sisters, is my rock, my source of strength, and my reason for fighting. Their unwavering support, their love, and their shared determination to overcome adversity have been a beacon of hope in the darkest of times. Together, we stand united in our quest for healing, for wholeness, and for a future free from the shadow of cancer.

And then there's my husband – my soulmate, my confidant, and my pillar of support. In him, I've found a kindred spirit, a partner who shares my dreams, my fears, and my unwavering faith in the power of love. Together, we navigate the twists and turns of this journey, drawing strength from each other and from the unbreakable bond that binds us together.

But perhaps the most compelling reason to fight is my 22-year-old son, who still needs me, who still looks to me for guidance, and who still believes in the possibility of miracles. He is my reason for waking up each morning with renewed determination, for facing each day with unwavering courage, and for refusing to let cancer define our future. In this battle, I draw inspiration from the countless stories of survival – tales of courage, resilience, and unwavering faith that serve as a beacon of hope in the darkest of times. These stories remind me that I am not alone, that there is strength in solidarity, and that together, we can overcome even the greatest of obstacles.

In the middle of the darkness, there is also light – the light of hope, of possibility, and of the promise of a brighter tomorrow. It's a light that shines through the cracks of despair, illuminating the path forward and guiding us towards a future filled with promise and potential.

As I continue on this journey, I'm reminded of the power of perspective – of the importance of focusing not on what might be, but on what can be. It's a mindset shift that empowers me to see beyond the confines of statistics and probabilities, and to embrace the infinite possibilities that lie ahead.

For me, faith isn't just a concept – it's a lifeline, a source of strength, and a light of hope in the darkest of times. It's the unwavering belief that no matter how dire the circumstances may seem, there is always a glimmer of hope on the horizon, a ray of light waiting to pierce through the darkness. I know that with God all things are possible.

And so, I speak life into existence – I declare that I will live and not die, that I will overcome this obstacle and emerge stronger and more resilient than ever before. It's a declaration of defiance, of resilience, and of unwavering faith in the power of the human spirit to overcome even the greatest of challenges.

But faith alone isn't enough – it must be accompanied by action, by a relentless pursuit of healing, and by a refusal to accept anything less than wholeness. It's a journey that requires courage, determination, and an unwavering commitment to self-care and self-love.

In this journey, I've come to realize that healing isn't just about the physical body – it's about nourishing the mind, body, and soul, and cultivating a sense of inner peace and well-being. It's about embracing practices that promote holistic health – from mindfulness and meditation to nutrition and exercise – and fostering a deep sense of connection with oneself and with the world around us.

But perhaps the most profound realization of all is that healing isn't a destination – it's a journey, a process of growth and transformation that unfolds over time. It's a journey that requires patience, perseverance, and an unwavering belief in the power of the human spirit to overcome even the greatest of challenges.

And so, I continue to press forward, one day at a time, one step at a time, trusting in the healing power of love, faith, and community to guide me towards a future filled with hope, possibility, and infinite potential. This battle is personal – but it's also a testament to the resilience of the human spirit, and the unbreakable bonds that unite us in our quest for healing and wholeness.

Despite not being diagnosed with cancer, I've encountered moments where the specter of the disease looms ominously over my life. I vividly recall a conversation from 16 years ago when someone cautioned me about the risks embedded in my bloodline, insinuating that my resemblance to my mother meant I was destined to face the breast cancer battle. It was a jarring encounter, one that initially unsettled me, but over time, I've learned to brush off such assumptions and instead focus on speaking life into existence.

For me, faith is paramount. It's the unwavering belief in the power of divine healing, a conviction that transcends the limitations of medical science. While others may place their trust in chemotherapy, radiation, or other treatments, I find solace in the knowledge that ultimate healing comes from a higher source. I've turned to prayer, beseeching God to cleanse my body of any lurking ailments, to shrink, expel, or eradicate anything that doesn't belong. My faith isn't just a passive belief; it's an active declaration of healing, a testament to the transformative power of faith.

In times of uncertainty, I find strength in the words of scripture – "By his stripes, I am healed." It's a reminder that healing isn't just a possibility; it's a promise, bestowed upon us through the ultimate sacrifice of Jesus Christ. And so, I continue to speak life, to declare victory over illness, and to trust in the divine plan that guides my journey. This battle may be personal, but my faith in God's healing power is unwavering, offering hope and reassurance in the face of uncertainty.

In the aftermath of that unsettling encounter, I found myself reflecting deeply on the power of words and the significance of perception in shaping our reality. While the words spoken to me were laden with fear and hurt I refused to let them define my destiny. Instead, I chose to reclaim my narrative, to speak life and abundance into existence, and to trust in the divine protection that surrounds me.

Over the years, I've come to understand that our beliefs have a profound impact on our physical and emotional well-being. By embracing a mindset of positivity and faith, we can cultivate an environment of healing and wholeness within ourselves. It's a transformative journey, one that requires courage, resilience, and an unwavering commitment to self-care and self-love.

In moments of doubt or uncertainty, I turn to prayer as a source of strength and guidance. I pour out my heart to a higher power, laying bare my fears and anxieties, and entrusting my health and well-being into His hands. It's a deeply personal connection, one that brings me comfort and solace in the midst of life's challenges.

And while I remain vigilant about my health, taking proactive steps to nurture my body and mind, I refuse to live in fear of what may or may not come to pass. Instead, I choose to focus on the present moment, embracing each day as a precious gift and an opportunity to live fully and authentically.

At the end of the day, the battle against breast cancer – or any form of illness – is not just a physical one; it's a spiritual journey, a testament to the resilience of the human spirit, and the power of faith to overcome even the greatest of obstacles. And so, I press forward with unwavering resolve, trusting in the healing power of God's love to guide me towards a future filled with hope, joy, and abundant life.

WHY SO YOUNG

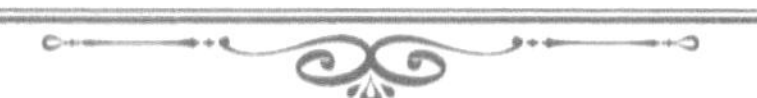

I have to be transparent; there are days when I question why my mother died so young. At the time, she didn't seem so young, but now that I am the exact same age, I realize she was very young. To die from breast cancer at 52, leaving behind a husband, seven children, and a granddaughter—I know my mother was not ready. She was scared. I remember praying with her, and even at the age of 26, I tried to pray fervently and earnestly to break through with a prayer. If I knew then what I know now, I would have fasted and prayed more. I would have been bolder at the throne of God. I would have recognized that at the age of 29, her mother died from ovarian cancer, leaving behind three daughters. I would have declared that they would live and not die.

I often wonder if it would have somehow made a difference, standing in the gap, exercising my faith for my mother. Could I have somehow covered her and petitioned the throne of God on her behalf for healing? Could I have somehow gotten my prayer through for complete healing?

Did the Lord grant my prayer and give her healing on the other side instead? I know He doesn't make mistakes; He is too wise to err. God is omniscient, omnipotent, and omnipresent, so He can't make a mistake. He knows the beginning to the end and the plans He has for us.

I remember my mother telling me that she had prayed and asked God to heal her, questioning if she had done something wrong to receive the fate of breast cancer. She told me she asked Him to heal her. God's ways are not our ways, and His thoughts are not our thoughts. We have to learn to trust Him and ask Him to give us the strength and the grace to accept His will for our lives.

I often find myself grappling with the weight of what could have been, questioning if my actions or prayers could have altered the course of my mother's journey. It's a burden that I carry with me, wondering if standing firm in faith, declaring healing, and pleading for mercy would have somehow changed the outcome. The echoes of those prayers, reverberating through the years, make me wonder if they reached the heavens or if they dissipated into the silence of my own desperation.

As I reflect on my mother's history, the tragic symmetry of her fate with that of her own mother adds another layer of complexity to my emotions. The premature loss of both these beautiful, young women to cancer, leaving behind a legacy of daughters, feels like a recurring nightmare. It's a familial thread woven with threads of sorrow, and I can't help but wonder if there is some cosmic lesson in this pattern or if it's simply the harsh reality of life's unpredictability.

In those moments of prayer, I yearned for a divine intervention, a miraculous healing that would defy the statistical odds stacked against her. The struggle to reconcile my belief in a merciful and all-powerful God with the harsh reality of her suffering is a conflict that lingers. Could my faith have been a catalyst for a different outcome, or was her destiny already written in the cosmic script?

The knowledge that God's ways are beyond human comprehension brings both solace and frustration. It is a paradox that demands acceptance and challenges the limits of our understanding. The strength to accept His will for our lives becomes a daily prayer, a plea for the wisdom to grasp the bigger picture, even when it remains elusive.

In retrospect, the realization that I cannot change the past forces me to confront the limitations of my humanity. The hindsight wisdom, the longing for a different outcome, and the hypothetical scenarios where I could have been more assertive in prayer all coalesce into a whirlwind of emotions that form the foundation of my grief.

Despite the unanswered questions and the lingering sense of what-ifs, I strive to find peace in the midst of this storm. I hold onto the belief that my mother's journey, though cut short, had a purpose that transcends the confines of my understanding. In the tapestry of life and death, faith and doubt, I seek a semblance of closure, embracing the mysterious ways in which God weaves the threads of our existence.

WOMEN ON THE BATTLEFIELD

Melissa Williams' journey is a testament to the human spirit's capacity for resilience and endurance. Despite facing numerous hurdles and setbacks, she remains undeterred, confronting each challenge with unwavering courage and grace. Her positive outlook and unwavering determination serve as a source of inspiration not only for those battling similar circumstances but for anyone navigating life's complexities.

Beyond her personal battle, Melissa's story resonates on a broader scale, shedding light on the importance of mental fortitude, faith, and the support of loved ones in overcoming adversity. Through her advocacy and willingness to share her experiences, she has become a beacon of hope and strength within her community, offering solace and encouragement to others facing similar trials.

In Melissa's presence, one cannot help but be uplifted by her infectious optimism and zest for life. Her resilience serves as a powerful reminder that even in the darkest of times, there is always a glimmer of hope to cling to. As she continues her journey, we stand in awe of her unwavering spirit and celebrate her triumphs, both big and small. Melissa W. is not just a survivor; she is a warrior, blazing a trail of resilience and hope for others to follow.

Despite Melissa's battle with breast cancer, she remains an awe-inspiring figure in the lives of those around her. As her friend, witnessing her journey has been both humbling and uplifting. Melissa embodies resilience, strength, and grace in the face of adversity, demonstrating the true essence of courage.

Throughout her ordeal, Melissa has never allowed her diagnosis to define her. Instead, she has continued to fulfill her roles as a devoted wife, loving daughter, nurturing mother, and loyal friend with unwavering determination. Despite the physical and emotional toll of her illness, she remains a pillar of unwavering strength for her family and friends.

One of the most remarkable aspects of Melissa's character is her unwavering faith in God. It is this faith that serves as her anchor, grounding her amidst the stormy seas of uncertainty and fear. Even in her darkest moments, she finds solace in her belief that there is a higher purpose guiding her through her journey.

In addition to her personal battles, Melissa is also a successful business owner. Her entrepreneurial spirit and creative talents have allowed her to thrive professionally, despite the challenges she faces on a daily basis. Her ability to channel her energy into her work serves as a testament to her resilience and determination.

Melissa's creativity knows no bounds. Whether she is designing intricate jewelry pieces, crafting beautiful works of art, or simply lending a listening ear to those in need, she approaches everything with a spirit of passion and dedication. Her talents not only enrich her own life but also bring joy and inspiration to those fortunate enough to know her.

Beyond her accomplishments and talents, it is Melissa's heart of gold that truly sets her apart. She is a compassionate soul who always puts the needs of others before her own. Her kindness knows no bounds, and she never hesitates to lend a helping hand or offer words of encouragement to those who are struggling.

As her friend, I am constantly in awe of Melissa's strength and resilience. She faces each day with unwavering determination and a smile on her face, refusing to let her illness dampen her spirit. Her positivity is contagious, and she has a knack for brightening even the darkest of days with her infectious laughter and unwavering optimism.

In the midst of her own battles, Melissa continues to uplift and inspire those around her. She is an example of hope and a shining example of the power of the human spirit to overcome even the greatest of challenges. Her journey is a testament to the strength of the human spirit and the transformative power of faith, love, and resilience.

Melissa is not just a survivor; she is a warrior, a beacon of hope, and a true inspiration to all who have the privilege of knowing her. Her unwavering faith, boundless strength, and compassionate heart make her a truly remarkable individual. I am beyond grateful to call her my friend, and I speak life and blessings over her as she continues her journey with courage and grace.

Connie F. Williams, just like Melissa and me, knows all too well the devastating impact of cancer. She's a breast cancer survivor who's been through her own share of battles. But what makes Connie's journey even more poignant is her personal connection to the disease. Like me, she lost her mother to cancer, so you can imagine the fear and uncertainty that must have gripped her when she received her diagnosis. I can relate to that feeling too; it's like history repeating itself, and the enemy whispering those dark thoughts in your ear.

On Connie's 59th birthday, of all days, the enemy tried to play mind games, reminding her that it was the same age her mother was when she passed away from cancer. It's like the universe was taunting her, trying to break her spirit. But Connie's made of stronger stuff. She didn't let that fear consume her. Instead, she faced her battle with grace and dignity, just like she does everything else in life.

Connie's faith has been her rock throughout this ordeal. It's what kept her going when everything seemed hopeless. She's a woman of deep conviction, and she's not afraid to speak life into her situation. She knows that despite the odds, there's always hope. And that's what she clings to, day in and day out.

What strikes me about Connie is her resilience. She's not one to broadcast her struggles; she faces them head-on, privately, without seeking pity or sympathy. But beneath that quiet strength lies a fierce determination to beat this thing. She's fought battles that most of us can't even imagine, and yet, she continues to soldier on with unwavering resolve.

Just like Melissa, Connie cherishes every moment, especially the time she gets to spend with her loved ones. She's not about to let cancer rob her of the joys of life. And while her journey may be filled with ups and downs, she faces it all with an indomitable spirit that's truly inspiring.

In the face of adversity, both Melissa and Connie exemplify what it means to have faith, courage, and resilience. They refuse to let cancer define them or dictate their future. Instead, they're writing their own story, one of hope, strength, and triumph over adversity. And in doing so, they're not just inspiring others; they're lighting the way for all of us to follow.

I must highlight the remarkable presence of Connie in our community. Connie is not just a friendly person; she is a leader, a voice, and a representation of hope for many. Her impact extends far beyond her immediate circle, reaching into the hearts and minds of those who seek inspiration and guidance.

Connie's leadership qualities are evident in every aspect of her life. Whether she is rallying support for a cause close to her heart or advocating for positive change within our community, she leads with integrity, compassion, and unwavering dedication. Her commitment to serving others is truly admirable, and she continues to inspire those around her to follow in her footsteps.

One of Connie's most notable achievements is her decision to run for public office was met with enthusiasm and support from the community, and it is no surprise why. Connie's passion for making a difference and her ability to connect with people on a personal level make her an ideal candidate for leadership roles. I hope that she continues to keep trying because the race is not given to the swift but to those who endure until the end.

In addition to her political endeavors, Connie is also a gifted speaker and emcee. Her infectious energy and vibrant personality have the power to captivate any audience, bringing life and vitality to every event she hosts. She has an awesome presence and style. Whether she is delivering a powerful speech or simply sharing a few words of encouragement, Connie's words have the ability to uplift, inspire, and motivate those around her.

Beyond her impressive resume and accomplishments, it is Connie's character that truly sets her apart. She is a woman of exceptional courage and strength, facing life's challenges with unwavering resolve and a positive attitude. Her resilience in the face of adversity serves as a source of inspiration for all who know her, reminding us that even in our darkest moments, there is always hope.

Connie's impact extends far beyond her individual achievements. She is a role model for many, a guiding light in times of darkness, and a voice for those who have none. Her advocacy for social justice and equality has touched the lives of countless individuals, empowering them to speak up and demand change. Through her actions and her words, Connie continues to make a lasting impact on our community, leaving behind a legacy of courage, compassion, and resilience.

Connie is more than just a leader; she is a force to be reckoned with, a true champion of the people, and a beacon of hope in a world that often feels uncertain. Her leadership, her passion, and her unwavering commitment to serving others make her an exceptional individual worthy of admiration and respect. I am honored to know Connie and I have no doubt that she will continue to inspire and uplift those around her for many years to come.

Donna's story is one of courage, resilience, and the power of friendship. For over three decades, she has been a constant presence in my life, a source of strength and inspiration through the ups and downs of life's journey. As a mother, wife, and friend, Donna has always been there for those she loves, selflessly giving of herself to uplift and support others.

Despite her private nature, Donna's recent battle with breast cancer has brought her story into the spotlight. Like a true warrior, she faced her diagnosis with unwavering determination and grace. When faced with the difficult decision of whether to undergo a double mastectomy, Donna approached it with courage and resolve, knowing that it was the best course of action for her health and well-being.

The decision to undergo such a major surgery is never easy, but Donna faced it head-on, knowing that it was a necessary step in her journey toward healing. Less than a month ago, she underwent the double mastectomy, a procedure that would change her life in ways she never could have imagined. Despite the physical and emotional toll of the surgery, Donna's spirit remained unbroken, her determination to overcome this obstacle unwavering.

As Donna navigates the challenging road to recovery, she does so with the support of her loved ones and the knowledge that she made the right decision for her health. In the weeks following her surgery, Donna has already returned to work, a testament to her strength and resilience. While the road ahead may be long and challenging, Donna faces it with optimism and hope, knowing that she has the love and support of her friends and family every step of the way.

The discovery of cancerous cells in her other breast only reinforces the importance of Donna's decision to undergo a double mastectomy. By taking proactive steps to remove both breasts, Donna has taken control of her health and significantly reduced her risk of recurrence. Her bravery in the face of adversity serves as an inspiration to us all, a reminder of the power of courage and determination in overcoming life's greatest challenges.

As Donna's friend, I am filled with admiration and gratitude for the incredible woman she is. Her strength, resilience, and unwavering faith are a testament to her character and her spirit. I am honored to stand by her side as she embarks on this journey of healing and recovery, offering whatever support and encouragement she may need along the way.

In the days, weeks, and months ahead, I speak life over Donna, praying for her speedy recovery and for her to enjoy life to the fullest. She is an amazing person, dear to my heart, and I know that she will emerge from this experience stronger and more resilient than ever before. With her unwavering spirit and the love and support of those who care for her, there is no doubt that Donna will overcome this obstacle and continue to inspire us all with her courage and grace.

Amy and Lauren's story. Breast cancer doesn't discriminate. It doesn't care about age, family history, or plans for the future. It can strike unexpectedly, shaking the very foundation of one's life. This harsh reality became evident when two of my closest friends, both in their early 50s, were diagnosed with breast cancer.

Both, vibrant and seemingly healthy, never anticipated facing such a formidable adversary. With no family history of the disease, they never worried about the possibility of breast cancer. Like many, they assumed it was a fate reserved for others, not themselves.

When the diagnosis came, it was a seismic shock. One opted for a double mastectomy, a decision marked by courage and strength. The other faced a different path, enduring rounds of chemotherapy and radiation alongside the removal of lymph nodes. Each treatment came with its own set of challenges, physical and emotional.

Witnessing their battles firsthand was a humbling experience. The resilience they displayed in the face of adversity was nothing short of extraordinary. Despite the fear and uncertainty, they confronted their diagnosis with unwavering determination. They refused to let cancer define them or dictate their future.

Throughout their journey, we rallied around them, offering unwavering support and encouragement. We spoke life into existence, refusing to succumb to the fear and despair that often accompanies such a diagnosis. Our bond grew stronger amidst the trials, a testament to the power of friendship and solidarity.

Early detection and screening played a crucial role in their recovery. It served as a reminder of the importance of proactive healthcare and regular check-ups. Their experiences underscored the significance of being vigilant and proactive when it comes to our health.

Today, both ladies are thriving. Their journey with breast cancer has transformed them in profound ways. It taught them resilience, gratitude, and the true value of life. They are living testaments to the power of hope, faith, and perseverance.

Their stories serve as beacons of hope for others facing similar battles. They remind us that even in our darkest moments, there is light to guide us forward. Breast cancer may have left its mark, but it did not dim their spirit or extinguish their hope.

As we celebrate their victories, we are reminded of the fragility of life and the resilience of the human spirit. Their journey is a testament to the power of community, support, and unwavering determination. It is a reminder that, together, we can overcome even the greatest of challenges.

The journey through breast cancer alongside two dear friends in their early 50s has been a profound testament to the resilience of the human spirit and the transformative power of faith. Witnessing their triumph over adversity has filled me with immense gratitude and awe. Knowing that they both emerged from this battle victorious brings a sense of relief and joy that is hard to put into words.

As someone who has not been diagnosed with cancer, I am acutely aware of the fragility of life and the uncertainty that accompanies it. The news of their diagnoses sparked a whirlwind of emotions within me - fear, uncertainty, and a deep sense of empathy for what they were facing. I couldn't help but contemplate the implications for my own health, considering the science, statistics, and familial history that often shape our perceptions of risk.

In the midst of my own unease, I turned to faith and prayer for solace and guidance. I refused to let fear dictate my response to their diagnoses. Instead, I chose to speak life into existence, denouncing any semblance of illness or disease that may seek to encroach upon our lives. I sent the specter of cancer to the pits of hell, invoking the power of faith to shield us from its grasp.

My belief in the power of declarations was strengthened as I witnessed their unwavering faith and determination. Despite the challenges they faced, they refused to be defined by their diagnosis. They embraced each day with courage and grace, trusting in a higher power to guide them through the darkest of times.

Their journey has reaffirmed my belief in the resilience of the human spirit. It has taught me that even in the face of seemingly insurmountable odds, hope endures. As I look to the future, I do so with optimism and resilience. I refuse to be defined by fear or uncertainty, choosing instead to walk in faith and confidence.

Breast cancer may cast its shadow, but it cannot extinguish the light of hope that burns within me. With faith as my guide, I am confident that I will overcome any obstacle that may come my way. And as I continue to stand alongside my friends, rejoicing in their victory, I am reminded of the words spoken by the psalmist: "I shall not die, but live, and declare the works of the Lord." These words resonate deeply within my soul, inspiring me to embrace life with gratitude and purpose.

Patti LaBelle is a name synonymous with talent, grace, and resilience. Though I've never had the privilege of meeting her in person, her presence in the world of music and entertainment has left an indelible mark on my life. From her angelic voice to her unwavering strength in the face of adversity, Patti LaBelle embodies the epitome of class and resilience.

Patti's remarkable career spans decades, marked by countless achievements and accolades. Her voice, with its soulful timbre and unmatched range, has captivated audiences around the world, earning her a place among the music industry's most iconic figures. But beyond her musical talent, it is Patti's spirit and character that truly set her apart.

Despite her immense success, Patti's life has not been without its challenges. Like many others, she has faced the devastating impact of cancer within her own family. The loss of several sisters to the disease is a heartbreaking reminder of the indiscriminate nature of illness and the fragility of life. Yet, through it all, Patti has remained steadfast in her resolve, refusing to let tragedy define her.

As someone who has also been told of a predisposition for cancer based on genetics and bloodline, I feel a sense of affinity with Patti. It's a reminder of the fragility of life and the importance of cherishing each moment we're given. But even in the face of such sobering realities, Patti's story serves as a beacon of hope and inspiration.

Despite the odds stacked against her, Patti continues to defy expectations, proving that her story doesn't have to follow the script written by science or statistics. Instead, she draws strength from her faith and the knowledge that she is not alone in her journey. Like so many others who have faced similar battles, Patti leans on the power of prayer and the support of her loved ones as she navigates the challenges of illness and recovery.

For those of us looking on from the sidelines, Patti's resilience is nothing short of awe-inspiring. She is a testament to the power of the human spirit to overcome even the greatest of obstacles, and her story serves as a reminder that there is always hope, even in the darkest of times.

As I speak life over Patti, I am filled with gratitude for the example she sets and the light she brings into the world. Her unwavering faith and resilience are a source of inspiration to us all, reminding us that with God, all things are possible. And though her journey may be marked by trials and tribulations, I have no doubt that Patti will emerge from this chapter of her life stronger and more resilient than ever before.

Patti LaBelle's story is not just one of survival, but of triumph. It is a testament to the power of faith, resilience, and the indomitable human spirit. And as we continue to follow her journey, we are reminded that even in our darkest moments, there is always hope, and that with God by our side, we can overcome any obstacle that comes our way.

Kathy Bates, much like Patti LaBelle, is a shining example of strength and resilience in the face of adversity. As an acclaimed actress, Kathy has graced the screen with her talent and charisma, captivating audiences with her unforgettable performances. But behind the glitz and glamour of Hollywood lies a story of courage and perseverance that is truly inspiring.

Throughout her career, Kathy has tackled a wide range of roles, showcasing her versatility and depth as an actress. From her Oscar-winning performance in "Misery" to her iconic roles in "Fried Green Tomatoes" and "Titanic," Kathy has left an indelible mark on the world of film and television. But perhaps her greatest role is the one she plays in her own life: that of a survivor. I must say she is one of my favorites. I absolutely loved her role in Fried Green Tomatoes, Titanic and A family that Preys.

In 2003, Kathy was diagnosed with ovarian cancer, a diagnosis that would forever change the course of her life. Like so many others facing a similar battle, Kathy was forced to confront the harsh realities of illness and mortality. But true to form, she refused to let cancer define her, choosing instead to face it head-on with courage and determination. Kathy's journey with cancer has been marked by both triumphs and setbacks. She underwent a double mastectomy and emerged from the experience with a renewed sense of purpose and gratitude for life. Throughout it all, she has been open and honest about her struggles, using her platform to raise awareness about ovarian cancer and the importance of early detection.

Despite the challenges she has faced, Kathy remains as vibrant and resilient as ever. She continues to pursue her passion for acting, refusing to let illness stand in the way of her dreams. Her unwavering spirit and determination serve as an inspiration to us all, reminding us that even in our darkest moments, there is always hope.

As I speak life over Kathy, I am filled with admiration for the incredible woman she is. Her strength, resilience, and unwavering faith are a testament to her character and her spirit. I pray for her continued health and well-being, knowing that she will emerge from this chapter of her life stronger and more resilient than ever before.

In the end, Kathy Bates' story is one of triumph over adversity, of resilience in the face of uncertainty. She is a beacon of hope and inspiration to all who know her, a reminder that with courage and determination, anything is possible. And as we continue to follow her journey, we are reminded that even in our darkest moments, there is always light, and that with faith and perseverance, we can overcome any obstacle that comes our way.

FAITH AND SCIENCE

As I sit down to reflect on my friends' journey with breast cancer, I am confronted with a mixture of emotions and thoughts. The journey has been arduous, marked by moments of fear, uncertainty, and profound introspection. Yet, amidst the turbulence, there has been a steadfast anchor that has guided me through the storm – my unwavering faith in God. God is my rock and my fortress. He is the reason for my being.

Science and doctors would assert that my familial history of breast cancer places me at a higher risk of succumbing to the same fate. Both my mother and her sister, my beloved aunt, fell victim to this relentless disease. The statistics would suggest that I am next in line, destined to battle the same adversary that claimed the lives of two of the most important women in my life. However, I have chosen to challenge the deterministic narrative that science paints.

In the face of daunting odds, I have made a conscious decision to denounce the limitations imposed by science alone. While I do not discount the invaluable contributions of medical research and the advancements made in the field of oncology, I firmly believe that ultimate healing transcends the realm of empirical evidence. My faith teaches me that healing is not solely contingent upon statistical probabilities or genetic predispositions; rather, it emanates from a divine source – God Himself.

Jehovah Rapha, the God who heals, is my beacon of hope in the midst of despair. His promises resonate deep within my soul, offering solace and assurance in moments of vulnerability. While some may view my reliance on faith as an act of defiance against scientific reasoning, I see it as a harmonious integration of both realms – faith and science.

Acknowledging the efficacy of medical interventions such as radiation, chemotherapy, and surgery does not negate my belief in the healing power of God. On the contrary, it reinforces the notion that God often works through tangible means to bring about miraculous outcomes. I am cognizant of the fact that my journey may necessitate undergoing rigorous treatments prescribed by medical professionals. However, my trust lies not in the efficacy of data and science, but in the overarching sovereignty of God.

Each thought of my mother serves as a poignant reminder of my mortality, yet it also serves as a testament to the resilience of the human spirit. God's presence envelops me, infusing me with a sense of peace that transcends understanding.

Throughout my early journey of fear and uncertainty, I have been surrounded by a network of unwavering support – family, friends, and fellow believers who have lifted me up in prayer and stood by my side in the darkest of times. Their love has been a tangible manifestation of God's grace, sustaining me through moments of weakness and doubt.

In the quiet moments of introspection, I find myself contemplating the intricate tapestry of life – its joys, sorrows, and everything in between. Breast cancer has forced me to confront my own mortality and reevaluate my priorities. It has taught me to cherish each moment, to embrace the beauty of imperfection, and to find gratitude in the midst of adversity.

As I navigate the twists and turns of this unpredictable journey, I am reminded of the words of the Psalmist: "Even though I walk through the darkest valley, I will fear no evil, for you are with me; your rod and your staff, they comfort me" (Psalm 23:4, NIV). Though the path ahead may be fraught with uncertainty, I take comfort in the knowledge that I am held securely in the palm of God's hand.

My journey rejecting and denouncing the fate of breast cancer has been a testament to the intersection of faith and science. While science may provide insights into the mechanisms of disease and offer avenues for treatment, it is faith that sustains me through the valleys of despair and carries me to the mountaintops of hope. I am grateful for the gift of life, for the opportunity to witness God's unfailing love in the midst of confronting fear. And so, I journey onward, guided by faith, sustained by hope, and enveloped in the enduring embrace of God's love.

In embarking on this narrative of my journey rejecting the fate of breast cancer, I feel compelled to steer away from the typical discourse of statistics, treatment modalities, and clinical prognostications. While such information undoubtedly holds its merit and importance, my intention is not to inundate the reader with facts and figures. Instead, I seek to delve into the profound intertwining of faith and science in the face of adversity.

Breast cancer, a formidable foe that has claimed the lives of countless women, has left an indelible mark on my family history. The loss of my mother and aunt to this relentless disease cast a long shadow of apprehension over my own journey. I choose to anchor myself in faith – faith in a God whose healing power transcends the confines of empirical evidence.

In a world where science often reigns supreme, the notion of coupling it with faith may seem incongruous to some. However, I firmly believe that the two are not mutually exclusive; rather, they can exist in harmonious tandem. Many medical professionals, in moments of candor, acknowledge that while they play a pivotal role in the treatment process, the ultimate healer is divine.

The sovereignty of God permeates every facet of my journey with breast cancer. His omnipotent hand guides the course of my treatment, infusing each step with purpose and meaning. While I am grateful for the advancements in medical science that afford me access to life-saving treatments, I am acutely aware that true healing emanates from a higher source.

Throughout the pages of Scripture, we are reminded of God's unwavering commitment to His children's well-being. The words of Isaiah resonate deeply within my soul: "But he was pierced for our transgressions, he was crushed for our iniquities; the punishment that brought us peace was on him, and by his wounds we are healed" (Isaiah 53:5, NIV). The sacrificial death of Jesus Christ serves as a beacon of hope, offering redemption and healing to all who believe.

I find solace in the promise that God's will shall prevail. Though the path ahead may be fraught with uncertainty, I take comfort in the knowledge that His plans are sovereign and His purposes unshakeable. The words of Jesus echo in my heart: "Your will be done, on earth as it is in heaven" (Matthew 6:10, NIV). Even in the face of adversity, I trust in the divine orchestration of events that unfolds according to His perfect will.

The concept of divine healing is not a mere abstraction; it is a tangible reality that permeates every fiber of my being. In the quiet moments of prayer, I am reminded of the balm in Gilead – a soothing salve that brings comfort and restoration to the weary soul. While medical treatments may alleviate physical symptoms, it is the healing touch of God that brings wholeness to the brokenhearted.

My journey serves as a testament to the profound interplay between faith and science. While I respect and acknowledge the invaluable contributions of medical professionals, I refuse to place my ultimate trust in human intervention alone. Instead, I choose to anchor myself in the unwavering faith that God is the ultimate healer – His will sovereign, His power unmatched. As I journey onward, I am reminded of the words of the Psalmist: "I lift up my eyes to the mountains—where does my help come from? My help comes from the Lord, the Maker of heaven and earth" (Psalm 121:1-2, NIV). Indeed, in Him alone do I find strength, hope, and healing.

In the midst of my own unease, I turned to faith and prayer for solace and guidance. I refused to let fear dictate my life.

Instead, I chose to speak life into existence, denouncing any semblance of illness or disease that may seek to encroach upon our lives. I sent the specter of cancer to the pits of hell, invoking the power of faith to shield us from its grasp.

The scripture "I shall not die, but live, and declare the works of the Lord" from the King James Version of the Bible became a mantra of hope and assurance during this tumultuous time. It served as a reminder that life is a precious gift, and that even in the face of adversity, there is hope for a brighter tomorrow.

I recalled the timeless wisdom that "the power of life and death is in the tongue." This biblical principle underscores the profound impact of our words and declarations. By speaking words of faith, healing, and life, we can shape our reality and overcome even the most daunting challenges.

I also found solace in the promise that "by the stripes of Jesus Christ, I am healed." This powerful declaration of healing served as a beacon of hope, reminding me of the redemptive power of Christ's sacrifice. Through his stripes, we find healing and restoration, both physically and spiritually.

Breast cancer may cast its shadow, but it cannot extinguish the light of hope that burns within me. With faith as my guide and the power of declarations on my lips, I am confident that I will overcome any obstacle that may come my way. And as I continue to stand alongside my friends, rejoicing in their victory, I am reminded of the enduring truth that faith, hope, and love conquer all.

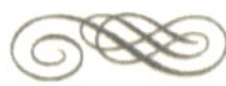

IN THE DEPTHS OF MY soul, I am convicted by the profound truth that God has bestowed upon me the extraordinary ability to speak things into existence. Through his word, He has given us all the ability through faith to speak over our lives. It is a divine gift, a manifestation of His boundless love and grace. Through the lens of faith, I perceive the world not merely as it is, but as it can be – a realm where miracles unfold at the sound of my voice. I know that I am special. I am an anointed woman of God. I am set aside. I am different. I belong to God and I profess Him to be my Lord and Savior. The power is not within me, but from God.

Scripture resonates within me, reinforcing this sacred truth. Romans 4:17 declares, "God, who gives life to the dead and calls those things which do not exist as though they did." In this verse, I find solace and empowerment. It is a testament to the limitless power of God, who speaks forth creation from nothingness. Just as He breathes life into the void, so too can I speak forth life into every corner of my existence.

The profound reality that life and death reside within the tongue is echoed in the wisdom of Proverbs 18:21: "Death and life are in the power of the tongue, and those who love it will eat its fruit." This scripture serves as a poignant reminder of the immense responsibility bestowed upon me. With each utterance, I hold the power to shape destinies, to sow seeds of abundance or destruction. Everyone who believes in the power of God has the same power. He gives this to all of us. Therefore, I choose life. I choose to infuse every word with the divine essence of hope, healing, and restoration.

In the sanctuary of prayer, I lift my voice with fervent conviction, speaking life into the very essence of my being. I declare with unwavering faith, "We shall live and not die, and declare the works of the Lord" (Psalm 118:17). These words resonate deep within my spirit, dispelling the shadows of doubt and despair. I declare and decree that the devil is a Liar and there is no truth in Him. I speak victory, a testament to the resilience of the human spirit when aligned with the divine.

Yet, I am acutely aware of the insidious presence of the enemy, seeking to ensnare me in the chains of generational curses. His whispers of death, sickness, and fear reverberate through the corridors of my mind, threatening to extinguish the flame of hope within me. But I refuse to succumb to his malevolent schemes. In the name of Jesus, I break every chain that binds me, every curse that seeks to imprison my soul (Galatians 3:13).

With unwavering faith, I declare the promises of God over my life and lineage. "I came that they may have life and have it abundantly" (John 10:10). These words are a beacon of hope, illuminating the path to wholeness and prosperity. Through the redemptive power of Christ's sacrifice, I am healed, my family is healed, my bloodline is healed (Isaiah 53:5).

As I navigate the turbulent waters of life, I am guided by the immutable truth that my words have the power to shape reality. With each declaration, I am sowing seeds of transformation, cultivating a harvest of blessings that transcends the confines of time and space. I am a vessel of divine light, an instrument of God's love and mercy in a world shrouded in darkness.

I know that the power of life and death resides within the tongue, a sacred trust bestowed upon me by a loving and merciful God. Through the lens of faith, I speak forth life into every aspect of my existence, declaring victory over every obstacle and adversity. With each word, I am forging a path to abundance, healing, and restoration, guided by the indomitable spirit of hope that resides within me.

I am but a humble servant, yet I am empowered with the divine authority to shape the course of my destiny and that of my loved ones. As I extend the mantle of my prayers and declarations, I am mindful of the countless souls who are battling with the burden of cancer. My heart aches for them, and in solidarity, I speak life into their bodies, minds, and spirits. I want everyone battling with cancer or everyone who doctors or science would say will battle this disease to know your power. I want to empower them to know that God is able to heal us. He is able to do things suddenly. He is able to do the impossible. We must believe it and we must speak it.

For those who are battling this insidious disease, I declare, "By His wounds, you are healed" (1 Peter 2:24). These words are a beacon of hope, a reminder that the healing touch of the Divine is ever-present, even in the darkest of nights. I envision a future where cancer is but a distant memory, where bodies are restored to wholeness, and spirits are infused with the radiance of divine light.

But my prayers extend beyond the confines of my immediate circle. They encompass all women who are dealing with the uncertainties of life, all those who are burdened by the weight of illness and despair. To them, I offer a message of hope and resilience, drawing inspiration from Isaiah 41:10: "Fear not, for I am with you; be not dismayed, for I am your God; I will strengthen you, I will help you, I will uphold you with my righteous right hand."

In the face of adversity, I stand unwavering, fortified by the promises of God and the indomitable power of faith. Though the road may be fraught with challenges, I am encouraged by the knowledge that I do not walk alone. With each step, I am accompanied by the guiding light of divine providence, leading me ever closer to the promised land of abundance and fulfillment.

As I reflect upon the journey that lies ahead, I am filled with a profound sense of gratitude. Gratitude for the gift of life, for the boundless love of a merciful God, and for the privilege of being a vessel of His grace. In the crucible of adversity, I have discovered the transformative power of faith, the enduring resilience of the human spirit, and the boundless depths of divine love.

I am reminded of the words of Jeremiah 29:11: "For I know the plans I have for you, declares the Lord, plans for welfare and not for evil, to give you a future and a hope." With these words etched upon my heart, I press forward, confident in the knowledge that God's promises are true, and His love endures forever. Through the power of faith and the spoken word, I shall continue to speak life into every corner of my existence, knowing that with God, all things are possible.

SEEKING THE GREAT PHYSICIAN

Enoch's story in the Bible has always captivated me. I've often pondered what it was about him that pleased God so much. There's something deeply intriguing about a man who walked so closely with the Divine that he bypassed death altogether. It's a mystery that stirs something within me—a longing to understand and emulate that kind of relationship with God.

I yearn to please God as Enoch did. I'm drawn to the idea of communing with Him, of talking to Him openly and honestly, just as Enoch did. If God found such delight in Enoch's heart and in his constant dialogue with Him, then surely that's the kind of relationship we're meant to have with our Creator.

Enoch's life serves as a compelling reminder that our relationship with God should be more than just religious rituals or occasional prayers. It should be a deep, meaningful connection—a friendship rooted in trust, love, and intimacy. Enoch's close relationship with God was evident in his daily walk with Him. He didn't just talk to God when he needed something; he spoke to Him constantly, sharing his joys, fears, and everything in between.

And God, in His infinite love and mercy, responded by bestowing upon Enoch a remarkable gift: exemption from death. It's a profound testament to the power of a life lived in close communion with the Divine—a life that pleases God beyond measure.

Enoch's story inspires me to cultivate a similar intimacy with God. I want to be known as someone who walks closely with Him, who seeks His presence in every moment, and who finds joy in simply being in His company. I want to pray fervently, not out of obligation, but out of a genuine desire to commune with my Heavenly Father.

In a world filled with distractions and busyness, it's easy to lose sight of what truly matters. But Enoch's life serves as a powerful reminder that our relationship with God should always be our top priority. It's in Him that we find true fulfillment, peace, and purpose.

As I reflect on Enoch's story, I'm reminded that God longs to have a personal relationship with each one of us. He delights in our presence, our prayers, and our love. And just as He did for Enoch, He longs to bestow upon us the gift of eternal life—a life lived in His glorious presence for all eternity.

In our journey of faith, we must strive to emulate the unwavering devotion and intimate communion that characterized the life of Enoch. His story serves as a poignant reminder of the transformative power of prayer and the profound impact of a life lived in constant communion with the Divine.

Enoch, a man of faith, walked so closely with God that he transcended the bounds of mortal existence. Genesis 5:24 recounts, "Enoch walked faithfully with God; then he was no more, because God took him away." This enigmatic verse speaks volumes about the depth of Enoch's relationship with the Almighty. He prayed fervently, communed intimately, and lived in alignment with the divine will.

Hebrews 11:5 attests to this remarkable testimony: "By faith Enoch was taken from this life, so that he did not experience death: 'He could not be found, because God had taken him away.' For before he was taken, he was commended as one who pleased God."

Enoch's life serves as a beacon of inspiration for believers across the ages. His example challenges us to cultivate a deeper intimacy with the Divine, to pray without ceasing, and to walk in unwavering faith. Like Enoch, we must approach the throne of grace with boldness and confidence, knowing that our prayers have the power to move mountains and shape destinies.

To truly experience the miraculous in our lives, we must approach God fervently and consistently. We must cultivate a spirit of relentless pursuit, seeking His face with unwavering determination and unyielding faith. Just as Enoch's persistent prayers moved the heart of God, so too can ours. James 5:16 affirms, "The prayer of a righteous person is powerful and effective."

Central to our faith journey is the fundamental belief in the omnipotence and benevolence of God. We must first believe that He is able and willing to intervene in our lives, to heal our bodies, mend our hearts, and restore our spirits. Hebrews 11:6 reminds us, "And without faith it is impossible to please God, because anyone who comes to him must believe that he exists and that he rewards those who earnestly seek him."

We must anchor our faith in the unchanging truth of God's Word. His promises are a testament to His faithfulness and unfailing love. John 10:10 declares, "The thief comes only to steal and kill and destroy; I have come that they may have life, and have it to the full." Through the sacrificial death of Jesus Christ on the cross, sickness, infirmity, poverty, and defeat were nailed to the cross. We have been given victory over every form of adversity and oppression because Jesus conquered it all.

As we journey through life, let us heed the timeless wisdom of Enoch's example. Let us pray without ceasing, commune intimately with the Divine, and walk in unwavering faith. In doing so, we will unlock the boundless blessings and miracles that await us, knowing that with God, all things are possible.

Enoch's story of walking closely with God is a profound testament to the transformative power of faith and prayer. His example challenges us to deepen our relationship with the Divine, to seek His presence with fervor and consistency, and to trust in His promises with unwavering faith.

In the hustle and bustle of daily life, it can be all too easy to lose sight of the importance of cultivating a vibrant prayer life and nurturing a close communion with God. Yet, Enoch's life serves as a compelling reminder of the extraordinary intimacy and profound spiritual depth that is attainable when we prioritize our relationship with the Divine above all else.

Philippians 4:6-7 exhorts us, "Do not be anxious about anything, but in every situation, by prayer and petition, with thanksgiving, present your requests to God. And the peace of God, which transcends all understanding, will guard your hearts and your minds in Christ Jesus."

Enoch's life underscores the importance of faith – not merely a passive belief, but an active, dynamic trust in the character and promises of God. Hebrews 11:6 reminds us that faith is the currency of heaven, the key that unlocks the door to divine favor and blessing. It is through faith that we lay hold of the abundant life that Christ came to give us, trusting in His unfailing love and providential care.

At the heart of our faith journey lies the unshakeable truth of God's Word. Just as Enoch walked in alignment with the divine will, so too must we anchor our lives in the timeless truths and promises contained within Scripture. Psalm 119:105 declares, "Your word is a lamp for my feet, a light on my path." As we meditate on God's Word day and night, it becomes a guiding light, illuminating our path and directing our steps.

In the scope of redemption, the sacrificial death of Jesus Christ on the cross stands as the ultimate expression of God's love and mercy towards humanity. Through His shed blood, we have been redeemed, reconciled, and restored to the right relationship with our Heavenly Father. 1 Peter 2:24 proclaims, "He himself bore our sins in his body on the cross, so that we might die to sins and live for righteousness; by his wounds you have been healed."

Indeed, the victory won on Calvary's hill is a victory that transcends time, space, and circumstance. It is a victory over sin, sickness, death, and every form of oppression that seeks to rob us of abundant life. As heirs of this victory, we are called to walk in the fullness of our inheritance, boldly declaring God's promises over our lives and standing firm in the assurance of His faithfulness.

The life of Enoch serves as a timeless testament to the transformative power of faith, prayer, and intimacy with God. His example challenges us to deepen our relationship with the Divine, to trust in His promises with unwavering faith, and to walk in the victory won for us on the cross. May we, like Enoch, be known as women who walk faithfully with God, communing with Him daily and trusting in His unfailing love.

Seeking the face of God, like Enoch, becomes a journey of healing, a journey where the belief in divine protection against sickness, against the encroachment of diseases like cancer, becomes a cornerstone of faith. Enoch's story, his walk with God so profound that he did not taste death, serves not merely as a biblical tale but as a beacon of hope, an exemplar of the possibilities within our grasp if only we dare to pursue the divine with all our hearts.

In our quest for health and wholeness, we echo Enoch's footsteps, seeking not just physical healing but a deeper communion with the Divine. It's a petition laid bare at the foot of the cross, a plea for the touch of Jesus to mend our bodies, to guard against the ravages of illness. But it's more than a transactional prayer for physical well-being; it's a cry for salvation, a desire to be held in the embrace of eternity by the hand of the Almighty.

Enoch's story is one of intimacy, of walking so closely with God that death itself dare not intrude. It speaks of a relationship beyond mere ritual, beyond rote prayers and empty gestures. It speaks of a genuine pursuit of the divine, a relentless seeking after the heart of God. And it's in this pursuit that we find not just healing but the promise of everlasting life.

For too long, perhaps, we've approached our faith as a transaction, a series of exchanges where we offer prayers in exchange for blessings, where we seek healing as if it were a commodity to be bought and sold. But Enoch's story challenges us to reframe our understanding of faith, to see it not as a means to an end but as an end in itself. It challenges us to seek God not for what He can do for us but for who He is, to pursue Him with the same fervor that drove Enoch to walk with Him for three hundred years.

And in this pursuit, we find healing of a different sort, a healing that goes beyond the physical to touch the very depths of our souls. It's a healing born of intimacy, of knowing and being known by the Divine. It's a healing that transforms us from the inside out, that fills the empty places within us with the presence of God.

But this healing, this communion with the Divine, is not just for our sake alone. It's a healing that spills over, that touches the lives of those around us. It's a healing that speaks to the brokenness of the world, offering hope where there is despair, light where there is darkness. It's a healing that points to the ultimate victory over sickness and death, a victory won on the cross of Calvary.

So let us, like Enoch, dare to seek the face of God, to pursue Him with all our hearts. Let us lay bare our souls at the foot of the cross, trusting in the healing touch of Jesus. And let us believe, with unwavering faith, that sickness will not overtake us, that cancer will not be victorious over our bodies. For if God was pleased with Enoch, if He walked with him so closely that death itself could not separate them, then surely He will be moved by our genuine pursuit of Him, by our petition for healing and salvation. And in the end, we will find not just healing but wholeness, not just health but eternal life in the presence of the Almighty.

SUPERNATURAL HEALING

I absolutely love the story of Hannah in the bible.

To truly seek the face of God, we must emulate the fervency of Hannah. Her story resonates with a raw, desperate longing for something seemingly out of reach—a desire for a child. In her anguish, she approached God with such intensity and emotion that she was mistaken for being drunk. But Hannah was not deterred; she boldly poured out her heart before the Almighty, knowing that He alone could grant her deepest desire.

In 1 Samuel 1:10-20, we see Hannah's heartfelt plea to God. She approached Him with everything she had, laying bare her soul in prayer. She knew that God had the power to intervene, to correct whatever was preventing her from conceiving a child. Like a skilled physician, she believed that God could heal her body and bless her with the gift of a child. Her prayer was not just a request for a baby; it was a plea for healing, for restoration, for the opportunity to bear fruit from her own body.

And God was moved by Hannah's approach. He heard her desperate cries and answered her prayers. In due time, Hannah conceived and gave birth to a son, Samuel, whom she dedicated to the service of the Lord. Her story is a powerful reminder that God responds to bold, fervent prayers, to those who seek Him with all their hearts.

In our own struggles with sickness and disease, we can draw strength from Hannah's example. We can approach God boldly, with the same intensity and desperation, knowing that He is the Great Physician who can heal our bodies and grant us total restoration. Just as He honored

Hannah's request for a child, He can honor ours for healing and wholeness.

When faced with the daunting prospect of cancer, it's easy to feel overwhelmed, to succumb to fear and despair. But Hannah's story reminds us that God is greater than any illness, that His power knows no bounds. He can block the hands of the enemy, thwarting every attempt to steal, kill, and destroy. He can turn our mourning into dancing, our despair into hope.

So let us, like Hannah, approach God with boldness and confidence, knowing that He hears our prayers and answers them according to His will. Let us pour out our hearts before Him, trusting in His unfailing love and mercy. And let us believe, with unwavering faith, that just as He healed Hannah and granted her request, He can do the same for us. For our God is a God of miracles, a God who delights in showing mercy to His children. And in His presence, there is healing, there is wholeness, there is hope.

Hannah's story not only demonstrates the power of fervent prayer but also the importance of surrendering our desires to God's will. Despite her deep longing for a child, Hannah vowed to dedicate her son to the service of the Lord if her prayer was answered. This act of surrender is a profound lesson for us all.

In our pursuit of healing, it's essential to align our desires with God's purposes. While we may desperately seek relief from sickness and pain, ultimately, our greatest desire should be to fulfill God's plan for our lives. Like Hannah, we must be willing to surrender our own desires and submit to God's perfect will, trusting that His plans are far greater than our own.

Surrendering to God's will doesn't mean giving up hope or resigning ourselves to suffering. Rather, it's an act of faith, a declaration that we trust God's wisdom and sovereignty, even when His plans don't align with our own. It's an acknowledgment that God's ways are higher than ours, and His timing is always perfect.

As we seek healing and restoration, let us follow Hannah's example of surrender and trust. Let us pour out our hearts before God, expressing our deepest desires and concerns, but also surrendering them to His loving care. And let us have faith that, just as God honored Hannah's surrender and answered her prayer, He will do the same for us.

In the midst of sickness and suffering, may we find comfort in knowing that we serve a God who is intimately acquainted with our pain, who hears our cries, and who is always working for our good. And may we take solace in the knowledge that, whether in sickness or in health, our ultimate healing and restoration are found in His loving embrace.

The Bible tells us plainly: Hannah couldn't conceive. It was a physical barrier beyond human remedy. But Hannah didn't resort to medical solutions or human interventions. Instead, she turned solely to prayer, believing God could achieve the impossible.

And He did. God heard her plea. He honored her request, miraculously opening Hannah's womb to bless her with Samuel, her son. It was a profound healing, defying logic and medical explanation.

What's truly remarkable is the simplicity of Hannah's healing. There were no surgeries, no medications, no elaborate treatments—just God's direct intervention. He remembered her, restoring her womb to perfect function. It's a powerful reminder that God is the ultimate healer, capable of defying all medical odds.

Hannah's story blesses my soul and gives me hope. It shows us that God's healing isn't bound by human limitations. Just as He answered Hannah's prayers and granted her a child, He can heal our sicknesses and restore us to health.

But Hannah's story isn't just about physical healing. It's about the potency of prayer, the strength of faith, and the beauty of surrendering to God's plan. It teaches us that even in our darkest hours, we can find solace in God's presence.

So, as we face illness and adversity, let's take comfort in knowing God hears our prayers. Let's trust that, like Hannah, He can answer our pleas and bring healing. Our God is a God of miracles, ready to extend His mercy and grace to His children. In His hands, there's healing, hope, and life.

Hannah's story isn't just about the natural order of things; it's a testament to God's supernatural power to intervene in our lives. Despite the physical impossibility of her situation, God blessed her supernaturally. Her barren womb became fertile, not through the workings of science or medicine, but through the direct intervention of the Divine.

This supernatural aspect of Hannah's story is crucial. It reminds us that God's blessings aren't limited by the constraints of the natural world. He operates beyond the boundaries of what we deem possible, performing miracles that defy logic and explanation.

Hannah's supernatural blessing offers profound hope. It's a reminder that God's healing isn't bound by the limitations of human understanding. I think it's so powerful when we understand that God can bless us supernaturally, transforming our circumstances in ways we never thought possible.

In our darkest hour, let's remember that God's blessings aren't confined to the ordinary. He can intervene supernaturally, bringing healing, restoration, and hope where there was once despair. Our faith isn't in the natural order of things, but in the supernatural power of the Almighty. When the doctors have said that there is no hope or the prognosis and diagnosis is not good, God is the great physician. He specializes in impossibilities. He can heal suddenly and instantly through the power of the holy ghost. If he chooses not to, it's not because he cannot do it. Just like He did for Hannah, He can heal supernaturally. We just have to ask and believe He can.

UNFORGIVENESS AND JEALOUSY

Jealousy, often described as a "green-eyed monster," has long been recognized as a corrosive force that can wreak havoc on both our psyche and physical well-being. Let me shed light on how jealousy rots the bones, as well as its profound implications for our mental and physical health.

I found scripture that offers profound wisdom on the destructive nature of jealousy. In the book of Proverbs, it is written, "A heart at peace gives life to the body, but envy rots the bones" (Proverbs 14:30, NIV). This metaphorical language paints a vivid picture of the insidious nature of jealousy. Just as bones provide structure and support to the body, a heart at peace sustains and nurtures life. However, envy, like a corrosive agent, eats away at the very foundation of our being, leaving us weakened and vulnerable. When I read this scripture, I couldn't help but be reminded of cancer.

You see, scripture equates jealousy with death itself, emphasizing its grave consequences. In the book of Song of Solomon, jealousy is described as "cruel as the grave" (Song of Solomon 8:6, NIV). This powerful imagery highlights the destructive power of jealousy, likening it to an unrelenting force that consumes everything in its path. Just as the grave signifies the end of life, jealousy symbolizes the death of relationships, happiness, and spiritual well-being.

Beyond its spiritual implications, jealousy also takes a significant toll on our mental health. I read that research has shown that envy is strongly associated with feelings of inadequacy, low self-esteem, and depression. When we constantly compare ourselves to others and covet what they have, we diminish our own sense of self-worth and happiness. This cycle of comparison and discontentment can spiral into a vicious cycle of negative emotions, leading to anxiety, stress, and even psychological disorders.

So, jealousy has tangible effects on our physical health. Chronic jealousy triggers the body's stress response, releasing hormones like cortisol and adrenaline into the bloodstream. While these hormones are essential for survival in threatening situations, prolonged exposure to stress hormones can wreak havoc on our bodies. Research has linked chronic stress to many health problems, including high blood pressure, heart disease, weakened immune function, and even accelerated aging.

Jealousy often leads to destructive behaviors that further compromise our physical well-being. In relationships, jealousy can manifest as possessiveness, control, and even violence. These toxic behaviors not only harm the individuals involved but also perpetuate cycles of abuse and dysfunction. Additionally, the emotional turmoil caused by jealousy can disrupt sleep patterns, appetite, and overall lifestyle habits, further exacerbating health problems.

In light of these profound insights, it becomes clear that jealousy is not only detrimental to our spiritual and mental well-being but also poses a significant threat to our physical health. As stewards of our own bodies and souls, it is incumbent upon us to recognize the toxic nature of jealousy and actively work towards its eradication. This requires cultivating a mindset of gratitude, self-compassion, and contentment, rather than succumbing to the pitfalls of comparison and envy.

Practicing mindfulness and gratitude can help reframe our perspective, shifting our focus from what we lack to what we have. By embracing a mindset of abundance rather than scarcity, we can cultivate a sense of inner peace and fulfillment that transcends external circumstances. I believe , nurturing healthy relationships built on trust, communication, and mutual respect can inoculate us against the corrosive effects of jealousy.

Also, the wisdom of scripture and my research converge to illuminate the destructive nature of jealousy and its profound implications for our well-being. From rotting the bones to being lower than the grave, jealousy exacts a heavy toll on our spiritual, mental, and physical health. To really get into what jealousy does to us, we've got to dig into why it happens in the first place. It's like this mix of feeling insecure, scared of losing something we care about, and not thinking much of ourselves. When we feel like our relationships, stuff, or status are at risk, our brains go into overdrive, and bam! Jealousy hits us like a ton of bricks.

Please understand that being jealous can seriously mess with our sleep, appetite, and overall vibe. Not getting enough sleep messes with everything, from our weight to our brain power. And being in a constant state of tension and worry can give us headaches, make our muscles all tense, and even mess with our stomachs.

So, how do we break free from the jealousy trap and get back to feeling good? It's all about getting real with ourselves, finding ways to cope, and surrounding ourselves with positive vibes. Talking it out with friends, family, or a pro can help us see things from a different angle and find ways to chill out. Plus, doing stuff like meditation, exercise, or creative stuff can help us relax and feel more balanced. We cannot afford to make ourselves sick.

And you know what else? We've got to change up how we see things. Instead of always comparing ourselves to others and feeling like we're missing out, let's focus on what's awesome about us. By celebrating our wins, big or small, and being grateful for what we've got, we can boost our self-esteem and feel way better about life.

I also say let's build up relationships that are all about trust, respect, and being real. When we've got folks in our corner who've got our backs, it's way easier to shrug off the jealousy and feel secure in who we are.

So yeah, jealousy might be a real pain, but we've got what it takes to kick it to the curb and live our best lives. It's all about finding our inner chill, focusing on the good stuff, and surrounding ourselves with awesome people who lift us up.

To delve deeper into the multifaceted nature of jealousy and its impact on our well-being, it's essential to understand the underlying psychological mechanisms that fuel this complex emotion. Jealousy often arises from a combination of insecurity, fear of loss, and low self-esteem. When we perceive a threat to our relationships, possessions, or status, our primal instincts are triggered, leading to feelings of jealousy and possessiveness.

Psychological research has identified two primary forms of jealousy: reactive and suspicious jealousy. Reactive jealousy occurs in response to a real or perceived threat to a valued relationship, such as infidelity or emotional betrayal. In contrast, suspicious jealousy arises from general mistrust and insecurity, leading individuals to constantly monitor their partner's behavior and suspect wrongdoing without evidence.

Both forms of jealousy can have detrimental effects on our mental and emotional well-being. Reactive jealousy often leads to intense emotional distress, anger, and resentment, which can strain relationships and erode trust. Suspicious jealousy, on the other hand, fosters a chronic state of anxiety and hypervigilance, undermining our ability to experience intimacy and connection with others.

Furthermore, jealousy is often accompanied by a host of cognitive distortions that reinforce negative beliefs about ourselves and others. These distortions, such as catastrophizing, mind-reading, and black-and-white thinking, perpetuate a cycle of irrational thoughts and behaviors that fuel jealousy. For example, someone experiencing jealousy may catastrophize a minor incident, believing it to be evidence of betrayal or abandonment.

Moreover, social comparison plays a significant role in exacerbating jealousy. In today's hyperconnected world, we are constantly bombarded with images and narratives of success, happiness, and perfection on social media platforms. This constant exposure to idealized versions of other people's lives can fuel feelings of inadequacy and envy, leading us to compare ourselves unfavorably and magnify our insecurities.

In addition to its psychological toll, jealousy can have profound physiological effects on the body. As mentioned earlier, chronic jealousy triggers the body's stress response, releasing a cascade of hormones that prepare us for fight or flight. While this response is adaptive in short bursts, prolonged exposure to stress hormones can lead to a host of health problems, including hypertension, cardiovascular disease, and compromised immune function.

Furthermore, the emotional turmoil caused by jealousy can disrupt our sleep patterns, appetite, and overall lifestyle habits, further compromising our physical health. Sleep deprivation, in particular, has been linked to a myriad of health issues, including obesity, diabetes, and cognitive decline. Additionally, the constant state of tension and anxiety associated with jealousy can lead to muscle tension, headaches, and other psychosomatic symptoms.

To break free from the grip of jealousy and reclaim our well-being, it's essential to cultivate self-awareness, emotional resilience, and healthy coping strategies. This may involve seeking support from trusted friends, family members, or mental health professionals, who can provide perspective, empathy, and guidance. Additionally, practicing self-care activities such as mindfulness meditation, exercise, and creative expression can help alleviate stress and promote emotional balance.

Moreover, developing a mindset of abundance and gratitude can counteract the scarcity mentality that fuels jealousy. By focusing on our own strengths, accomplishments, and blessings, we can cultivate a sense of self-worth and fulfillment that transcends external comparisons. Building meaningful connections based on trust, respect, and authenticity can also foster a sense of security and belonging that mitigates jealousy.

I believe that jealousy is a complex and pervasive emotion that makes people sicker than they realize. From its roots in insecurity and fear to its manifestation in cognitive distortions and physiological stress, jealousy permeates every aspect of our lives. However, by cultivating self-awareness, resilience, and healthy coping strategies, we can transcend the grip of jealousy and embrace a life of wholeness, connection, and fulfillment.

Unforgiveness really takes its toll on our health, you know? It's like this weight that we carry around, dragging us down physically, mentally, and emotionally. I've read somewhere about how holding onto grudges can actually affect your well-being, and it totally makes sense. It's not just some abstract concept; it's something that manifests in our bodies and minds.

I remember coming across this scripture that really hit me hard. It talked about how God won't forgive us until we forgive others. At first, it seemed kind of harsh, you know? But the more I thought about it, the more it made sense. It's like this divine exchange—our forgiveness of others mirrors God's forgiveness of us. It's almost like a prerequisite for receiving that forgiveness.

But it's not just about some divine transaction; it's about freeing ourselves from the chains of resentment and bitterness. Harboring unforgiveness is like locking ourselves in a prison of our own making. It keeps us stuck in the past, unable to move forward. And it's not just about forgiving others; it's also about forgiving ourselves. We all make mistakes, we all fall short, and we all need forgiveness—daily, even.

I've come to realize that forgiveness isn't just a one-time thing; it's a daily practice. It's about letting go of the hurt and the pain, over and over again if necessary. It's about choosing to release the grip that those past offenses have on us and embracing the freedom that comes with forgiveness.

And you know what's really crazy? The more I've leaned into forgiveness, the lighter I've felt. It's like this burden has been lifted off my shoulders, and I can finally breathe again. It's not easy, don't get me wrong. There are days when I still struggle with feelings of resentment and anger. But I've learned that forgiveness isn't about denying those feelings; it's about acknowledging them and then choosing to let them go.

I think that's what's so beautiful about forgiveness—it's a choice. We have the power to choose whether we want to hold onto bitterness or whether we want to embrace freedom. And yeah, it's scary sometimes, stepping into that unknown territory of forgiveness. But it's also incredibly liberating.

So yeah, unforgiveness definitely has its toll on our health, both physically and spiritually. But the good news is that we don't have to stay stuck in that place of bitterness and resentment. We have the power to choose forgiveness, to choose freedom, and to choose healing. And that's something worth holding onto.

Unforgiveness is like a roadblock on the path to healing and wellness, and let me tell you, it's a hefty one. When we hold onto grudges, resentment, and bitterness, we're essentially locking ourselves in a cycle of pain and suffering. It's like we're trapping ourselves in this negative energy that not only affects our emotional and mental well-being but also takes a toll on our physical health.

Let's break it down a bit. When we harbor unforgiveness, our bodies are flooded with stress hormones like cortisol. This prolonged state of stress can be very hard on our immune system, making us more susceptible to illness and disease.

But it's not just our physical health that takes a hit—it's also our mental and emotional well-being. Holding onto unforgiveness can lead to feelings of anger, resentment, and even hatred. These negative emotions can consume us, eating away at our happiness and peace of mind. It's like we're carrying around this heavy burden, weighing us down and preventing us from experiencing true joy and fulfillment.

And let's not forget about the impact unforgiveness has on our relationships. When we're unable to forgive others, it creates this barrier between us and them. It's like we're building walls instead of bridges, isolating ourselves from the people around us. This lack of connection can lead to feelings of loneliness and isolation, further exacerbating our emotional pain.

But here's the thing: forgiveness isn't just about letting go of the past; it's also about reclaiming our power. When we forgive others, we're not saying that what they did was okay; we're saying that we refuse to let their actions define us. We're choosing to take back control of our lives and move forward with grace and compassion.

And here's where the magic happens—when we choose forgiveness, we open ourselves up to healing and transformation. It's like we're removing that roadblock and allowing the energy of healing to flow freely through us. We're creating space for love, joy, and peace to enter our lives, replacing the darkness of unforgiveness with the light of healing.

But make no mistake, forgiveness is not always easy. It requires courage, vulnerability, and a willingness to let go of our ego. It means confronting our pain head-on and choosing to release it, even when every fiber of our being wants to hold onto it. But the rewards are worth it—freedom from pain, peace of mind, and a renewed sense of purpose and vitality.

So if you're struggling with unforgiveness, know that you're not alone. It's a journey, and it's okay to take it one step at a time. Reach out for support if you need it—whether it's through therapy, counseling, or simply talking to a trusted friend. And remember, the power to heal lies within you. You have the ability to break free from the chains of unforgiveness and embrace a life filled with love, joy, and well-being.

Jealousy and unforgiveness are like toxic weeds in the garden of our souls, choking out the beautiful flowers of love, joy, and peace. And let me tell you, they don't just wither away on their own; they fester and grow, spreading their poison throughout our entire being. It's like a disease that infects every aspect of our lives, from our relationships to our physical health.

You see, jealousy and unforgiveness are not just harmless emotions; they're deadly weapons that can destroy us from the inside out. When we allow jealousy to take root in our hearts, it eats away at our self-esteem and erodes our trust in others. We become consumed by comparison, constantly measuring ourselves against others and feeling inadequate as a result.

And then there's unforgiveness—the silent killer of the soul. When we hold onto grudges and resentments, we're essentially drinking poison and expecting the other person to die. It's like we're carrying around this heavy burden, weighed down by the pain of the past. And the longer we hold onto it, the heavier it becomes, until it eventually crushes us under its weight.

But here's the thing: we were never meant to carry that burden alone. We were never meant to navigate the treacherous waters of jealousy and unforgiveness without help. That's where Jesus Christ comes in. He is the ultimate healer, the one who can take our brokenness and turn it into something beautiful.

But here's the catch: we have to ask for his help. We have to invite him into our hearts and surrender our jealousy and unforgiveness to him. It's not enough to just acknowledge their presence; we have to actively seek their removal from our lives.

And here's the good news: Jesus is more than willing to help us. In fact, he's just waiting for us to ask. He longs to heal our brokenness and set us free from the chains of jealousy and unforgiveness. But we have to be willing to let go of them—to release our grip and trust him to take care of the rest.

But make no mistake, overcoming jealousy and unforgiveness is not easy. It requires humility, vulnerability, and a willingness to let go of our pride. It means acknowledging our weaknesses and surrendering them to a power greater than ourselves. But the rewards are worth it—freedom from jealousy and unforgiveness, peace of mind, and a renewed sense of purpose and joy.

And here's the thing: it's not just about us. When we allow jealousy and unforgiveness to take root in our hearts, it affects everyone around us. It poisons our relationships, sowing seeds of discord and division. It damages our physical health, weakening our immune system and leaving us vulnerable to illness and disease.

So while we're asking God to heal us and preserve our bodies—our temples—we must also make sure to rid our temples of these toxic weeds that could aid in our destruction. We must ask Jesus to remove jealousy and unforgiveness from our lives daily, surrendering them to him and trusting him to replace them with love, joy, and peace.

Because here's the truth: jealousy and unforgiveness can actually kill us. They can rob us of our health, our happiness, and even our lives. But with Jesus by our side, we have the power to overcome them—to break free from their grip and embrace a life filled with hope, healing, and wholeness.

I have provided these scriptures for you on your journey of total forgiveness and a clean heart because they emphasize that forgiveness is not just a suggestion but a commandment for believers. It's not only about extending grace to others but also about aligning our hearts with the forgiveness we've received from God. Failure to forgive others can hinder our own experience of God's forgiveness and hinder our relationship with Him.

Matthew 6:14-15 (NIV): "For if you forgive other people when they sin against you, your heavenly Father will also forgive you. But if you do not forgive others their sins, your Father will not forgive your sins."

Mark 11:25-26 (NIV): "And when you stand praying, if you hold anything against anyone, forgive them, so that your Father in heaven may forgive you your sins."

Colossians 3:13 (NIV): "Bear with each other and forgive one another if any of you has a grievance against someone. Forgive as the Lord forgave you."

Ephesians 4:32 (NIV): "Be kind and compassionate to one another, forgiving each other, just as in Christ God forgave you."

Luke 17:3-4 (NIV): "So watch yourselves. If your brother or sister sins against you, rebuke them; and if they repent, forgive them. Even if they sin against you seven times in a day and seven times come back to you saying 'I repent,' you must forgive them."

Matthew 18:21-22 (NIV): "Then Peter came to Jesus and asked, 'Lord, how many times shall I forgive my brother or sister who sins against me? Up to seven times?' Jesus answered, 'I tell you, not seven times, but seventy-seven times.'"

Matthew 5:23-24 (NIV): "Therefore, if you are offering your gift at the altar and there remember that your brother or sister has something against you, leave your gift there in front of the altar. First go and be reconciled to them; then come and offer your gift."

SPEAK LIFE OVER YOURSELF

Speaking life over ourselves and our circumstances is a powerful practice that aligns with the principles of faith and spiritual well-being. When we speak positively over our health, our bodies, and our lives, we are essentially affirming our trust in God's promises and activating the power of faith to bring about positive change.

One of the foundational aspects of speaking life is acknowledging the authority of God's Word in our lives. Scripture tells us that "death and life are in the power of the tongue" (Proverbs 18:21), emphasizing the profound impact our words can have on our reality. By aligning our words with the truth of God's Word, we can declare healing, restoration, and wholeness over every aspect of our being.

When facing health challenges, it's crucial to speak declarations of health and healing over our bodies. We can declare that we will live and not die, affirming God's promise of abundant life for His children (John 10:10). We can declare that our bodies and health will align with the Word of God, trusting in His power to bring about supernatural healing and restoration.

It's essential to confess any sins or areas of unrighteousness in our lives and ask for God's forgiveness and cleansing. Scripture assures us that "if we confess our sins, he is faithful and just to forgive us our sins and to cleanse us from all unrighteousness" (1 John 1:9). By humbling ourselves before God and seeking His forgiveness, we open the door for His healing and transformational work in our lives.

Praying for God's intervention and supernatural healing is an integral part of speaking life. We can ask God to remove anything in our bodies that should not be there, including sickness, disease, or any form of illness. We can petition God to heal our bodies and minds, restoring us to health and wholeness according to His will.

This is something I firmly believe in. Seeking support from a prayer partner or community of believers is also encouraged in Scripture. Jesus Himself said, "Where two or three are gathered in my name, there am I among them" (Matthew 18:20). When we come together in agreement and unity, our prayers are strengthened, and God's presence is magnified in our midst. Having a prayer partner to touch and agree with us amplifies the power of our prayers and reinforces our faith in God's ability to heal and restore.

In addition to praying collectively, maintaining a personal relationship with God through daily communion and prayer is vital for spiritual growth and well-being. Scripture exhorts us to "pray without ceasing" (1 Thessalonians 5:17), emphasizing the importance of ongoing communication with God. By staying connected to God through prayer and fellowship, we cultivate a deeper intimacy with Him and experience His transformative power in our lives.

Ultimately, speaking life over ourselves and our circumstances is not just a mere exercise in positive thinking; it's a profound expression of faith and trust in God's sovereignty and goodness. As we align our words with God's Word, confess our sins, and petition Him for healing and restoration, we position ourselves to receive His abundant blessings and walk in the fullness of His promises.

These scriptures are very powerful and they affirm the power of our words to shape our reality and bring about transformation in our lives. By speaking God's Word and His promises in faith, we can declare healing, restoration, and victory over every circumstance we face. We must be intentional about our quest and our pursuit to healing and covering on a daily basis.

Proverbs 18:21 (NIV): "The tongue has the power of life and death, and those who love it will eat its fruit." This verse underscores the significance of our words in shaping our reality. Speaking words of life brings about positive outcomes, while words of death can have detrimental effects.

Mark 11:23 (NIV): "Truly I tell you, if anyone says to this mountain, 'Go, throw yourself into the sea,' and does not doubt in their heart but believes that what they say will happen, it will be done for them." Jesus emphasizes the power of faith-filled words to bring about miraculous outcomes, illustrating the importance of speaking in alignment with belief.

Romans 10:9-10 (NIV): "If you declare with your mouth, 'Jesus is Lord,' and believe in your heart that God raised him from the dead, you will be saved. For it is with your heart that you believe and are justified, and it is with your mouth that you profess your faith and are saved." Confessing and declaring our faith verbally is a foundational aspect of Christian belief and salvation.

Psalm 107:20 (NIV): "He sent out his word and healed them; he rescued them from the grave." This verse highlights the healing power of God's Word. When we speak God's promises of healing and restoration, we activate His supernatural intervention in our lives.

Isaiah 55:11 (NIV): "So is my word that goes out from my mouth: It will not return to me empty, but will accomplish what I desire and achieve the purpose for which I sent it." God's Word is powerful and effective, and when we speak

His promises in faith, they will not return void but will bring about the intended results.

2 Corinthians 4:13 (NIV): "It is written: 'I believed; therefore, I have spoken.' Since we have that same spirit of faith, we also believe and therefore speak." This verse underscores the connection between belief and confession. As believers, we speak in alignment with our faith in God's promises.

Matthew 12:36-37 (NIV): "But I tell you that everyone will have to give account on the day of judgment for every empty word they have spoken. For by your words you will be acquitted, and by your words you will be condemned." Jesus emphasizes the accountability we have for our words and the significance of speaking in alignment with righteousness.

Say this prayer daily. I pray that you are healed in the name of Jesus.
Dear Heavenly Father,

I come before you lifting up those who are battling cancer and those who carry the burden of predisposition to this illness. In my prayer, I speak words of life into their journey of healing. Lord Jesus I believe in your power to bring about restoration and renewal. I speak that we shall live and not die. In the mighty name of Jesus. Heal us or Jehovah Rapha!

Dear Lord please grant strength and comfort to those who are fighting this battle, and may your healing touch be upon them. I trust in your divine wisdom, knowing that even if healing does not come in the way we expect, it is not because of any limitation on your part. Help me to surrender to your will, accepting it with grace and understanding.

I turn to you, the Great Physician, seeking your guidance and intervention. Let your light shine upon me, dispelling the darkness of illness and despair. I declare with faith that I will live and not die, breaking the chains of generational curses and declaring your glorious works.

May your love surround me , bringing hope and comfort in my time of need. In your name Lord Jesus, I pray. Amen."

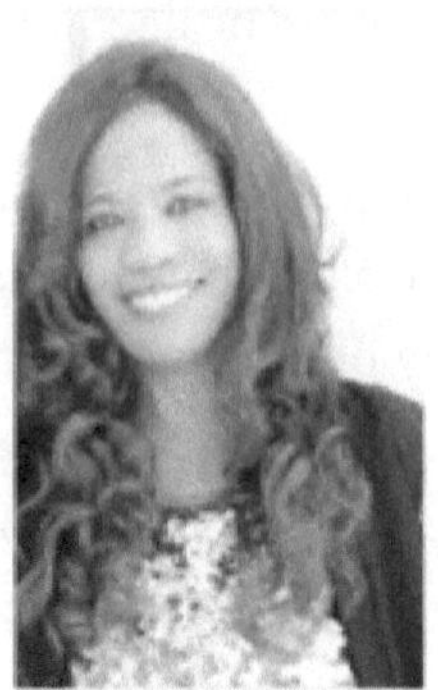

Meet The Author

Kim Ruff Moore is an acclaimed Stellar Award-winning singer, songwriter, and national recording artist, known for her soul-stirring performances as a member of the renowned group, The New Consolers. Beyond her musical talents, Kim is a dynamic author, speaker, and emerging authority in the realm of self-help advice for relationships and finances.

With a passion for empowering others, Kim's written works offer practical insights and spiritual wisdom to navigate life's challenges. Her diverse range of titles, including "Cuffed," "Never Place All Your Eggs In One Basket," "Serendipity," "Superheroes Teach," Jealousy Makes You Sick, Marriage Releases God's Favor and "Waymaker," reflect her multifaceted approach to personal growth and transformation.

As a Christian author, Kim infuses her writing with biblical principles and heartfelt encouragement, inspiring readers to cultivate healthy relationships, manage finances wisely, and deepen their faith. Through her engaging speaking engagements and meaningful content, Kim is dedicated to creating a positive impact and guiding individuals towards a more fulfilling life.

Kim Ruff Moore's powerful combination of music, literature, and motivational speaking underscores her commitment to uplifting others and spreading a message of hope and resilience. With her unique blend of talent and insight, she continues to inspire audiences across the globe, leaving a lasting imprint on hearts and minds alike.

Contact Email: Theprolificauthor@gmail.com

478-443-9468 Contact Number

BIBLIOGRAPHY

Ruff-Moore, Kim. *I Speak Life: Seeking The Great Physician.* Ruff-Moore Media, 2024.

And here are the cited scripture sources:

- Matthew 6:14-15 (NIV)
- Mark 11:25-26 (NIV)
- Colossians 3:13 (NIV)
- Ephesians 4:32 (NIV)
- Luke 17:3-4 (NIV)
- Matthew 18:21-22 (NIV)
- Matthew 5:23-24 (NIV)
- James 5:16 (NIV)
- Psalm 103:2-3 (NIV)
- 1 Peter 2:24 (NIV)
- Isaiah 53:5 (NIV)

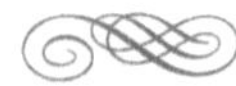

I SPEAK LIFE

Seeking the Great Physician

www.ingramcontent.com/pod-product-compliance
Lightning Source LLC
Chambersburg PA
CBHW021746150726
47989CB00004B/1534